What is Ketogenic Diet?

A ketogenic diet is a special form of diet is similar to a low carb diet, which results in the body into fat burning machine. The ketogenic diet is very helpful in treatment of many diseases like diabetes , ellipses and sometimes even in treatment in cancer.

The one on of the benefit of ketogenic diet is it can drastically help in reducing body weight, but it has also some potential drawback and side effects.

 In simple language, a ketogenic diet is a type of diet in which carbohydrates intake is low like 2-4% of calories. While the protein intake is high.

In this book, you will discover how to use ketogenic diet and mistakes to avoid during the ketogenic diet.

How ketogenic diet works?

Generally, when carbohydrates are converted into blood sugar it results into high blood pressure and high sugar level in the blood.

When we restrict the intake of carbohydrates and only eat protein and fat then there is a shift in our metabolic food processing.

Now since our body doesn't get enough amount of sugar(glucose i.e energy) in the form of carbohydrates so it starts depending on excess fat in our body. As a result, more fat is burned from our body .

When fat is burned it convert into a compound called Ketones. Also since the carbohydrates intake is stopped so the blood sugar level and insulin level are lowered. Since the insulin level falls and energy is required, so fatty acid flows from the fat cells into the blood stream.

Glucose is the main source of fuel for our body when the diet is high in carbohydrates, but when the carbohydrates are restricted ketone body becomes the main source of fuel in our body.

This is how Ketogenic diet works.

Benefits of Ketogenic Diet

According to medical research Ketogenic diet is responsible for the cure of many medical conditions as discussed below:

Cancer: Ketogenic diet is helpful in treatment of cancer the idea behind the treatment is to starve the cancer cells and provide support for the normal mitochondrial tissues. But the subject of the treatment of cancer is totally different from the subject of weight loss.

Diabetes: Ketogenic diet is helpful in maintaining the blood sugar level in our body and hence is very helpful in the treatment of diabetes. Again this is a totally different subject and in this book we will be discussing the cure of weight loss only.

Alzheimer's disease: Ketogenic diet is a helpful treatment of Alzheimer's disease as it helps in providing the necessary energy to brain.

Also, there have been many resources and research which shows that Ketogenic diet is helpful in the treatment of the following health conditions also.

The information provided herein is stated to

Heart disease, Autism, Neurological disorders, Aging is slowed.

And much more.

Facts about Ketogenic diet which you didn't know

There have been many talks around the subject of ketogenic diet , many experts believe that ketogenic diet is not good for health and many believe that this diet can cause many side effects and result in many another type of diseases.

In this section you will discover those myths and learn the real facts about the ketogenic diet. These facts are based on the scientific research.

Misconception 1 : Carbs are necessary for good health

some people believe that carbohydrates are necessary to provide glucose to fuel brain. However, it is not necessary that carbohydrates are only the essential nutrients needed for the body. There are essential fatty acids and essential proteins but there is no essential carbohydrate.

When the body is in ketosis stage our brain switches to using ketone bodies to use necessary fuel needed, and less glucose is required as ketone bodies are used as an alternative fuel.

Our liver can make the necessary glucose needed for the brain from glycogen stored in the liver.

if the glucose is needed more by the body then the body can make glucose from the protein using the food.

It has been found that people in Africa and many other places live without carbohydrates.

So we can conclude carbohydrates are not mandatory nutrients for our body.

Misconception 2 Ketosis is dangerous for our body

Ketosis is entirely different term, ketosis is not dangerous but Ketoacidosis is

Ketosis- ketosis is an energy state when there is a glucose deficiency in body in this case our body provide an alternative fuel to our body by providing additional glucose to body. This happens when our body is in fasting state or starving state.

in general body cells metabolizes food nutrient and oxygen during respiration process. Most of this energy is produced in mitochondria. however there are two types of food based fuel from which our cells can produce energy.

1st type from cellular fuel: In this type of fuel production our body produces fuel from blood sugar also know as carbohydrates. a normal human body can store about 1000-1600 calories of glucose in the form of glycogen in our liver.

2nd Type of fuel: This type of fuel comes from fat as ketone bodies . On an average human body can store thousands of calories which is in the form of fat. Once our body is in starvation state then our body starts to burn fat in the form of fuel and hence starts to lose weight.

our brain and nerve cells can utilize the ketone when the glucose is not available. also our cells can produce much cleaner energy as the ketone bodies produce much cleaner fuel. also the cells create larger energy in case of ketosis than it can produce from normal glucose.

on the other hand ketoacidosis is different from ketosis. Many people confuse ketosis with ketoacidosis the difference is explained below-

- nutritional ketosis is a controlled, insulin-regulated process which results in mild release of fatty acids.
- Ketoacidosis on the other hand is caused by the lack of insulin in the body. due to which blood sugar level rises and as a result excess amount of fat burning results in large quantities of ketones. This in turn imbalances the normal acid/base balance in the blood and it turns out to be dangerous.

So to conclude, ketosis is not dangerous but ketoacidosis is dangerous for health.

Misconception 3. Kidney gets damaged from high consumption of protein

First of all ketogenic diet are not high protein diet but high-fat diet, in addition to little amount of protein consumption. so we can conclude that ketogenic diet is not harmful to our kidney.

Misconception 4. Ketogenic diet results in osteoporosis.

Osteoporosis occurs when there is large consumption of protein, due to which our body excrete calcium and result in osteoporosis. But as discussed above ketogenic diet is not high protein diet so there is no chance of osteoporosis.

Misconception 5 Ketogenic diet can cause in the development of heart diseases.

According to a study, a ketogenic diet like low carb diet eliminates the heart diseases makers in our body.

According to another study ketogenic diet blood result is favorable in the case of heart disease.

Also, many studies show that ketogenic diet is responsible for good vascular health and result in faster weight loss.

On the other hand, a study has shown many times that other high carbohydrates diet are responsible for heart diseases.

.

Misconception 6 Ketogenic diet causes muscle loss.

In reality, low carb diet are better at preserving lean muscle and also helps in increasing lean mass muscle.

on the other hand mass muscle can lose if the diet is high carb and insulin and blood sugar are high and no ketone body is present to fuel the brain.

Misconception 7 Ketogenic diet causes water loss and is not real

It is a fact that lowering the carbohydrate intake can result in water loss and but this is not permanent loss.

after few weeks our body adapts to its state of ketogenic state and the water loss reduces. However the water loss can be stabilized by taking 5g of potassium and magnesium per day in your diet.

Misconception 8 Weight will come back after you are off the low carb diet

this fact is true. if you want to remain lean always then you need to maintain the low carb diet everytime.

This is a body metabolic process which you are altering, you need to maintain the body metabolic process if you want to remain lean all the time. Switching back to the high carb diet will switch your body to the previous metabolic state and hence you will again start to gain weight.

Misconception 9 Ketogenic diet are low in fiber

This is not true as ketogenic diet includes lots of fibrous vegetables as we will discuss in the later section of this book. Ketogenic diet comes with fibrous vegetables like spinach, salads which are allowed in low carb diet.

Ketosis

Ketosis is nothing but an energy state when there is low is the availability of glucose and our body uses something called ketosis to provide the energy necessary for our body. This state is achieved when our body is in low energy state or when our body goes through the fasting state.

When we eat low carb and high fat this process enhances and the ketosis process gets to come into play.

As discussed above our body makes something called ketones bodies from stored fat

So how does this process takes place?

In order for our body to access the stored fat the blood sugar and insulin level should be low.

Now if your body has low blood sugar level and insulin level then this process happen to start, first, the stored fat also known as triglyceride. An agent called hormone sensitive lipase (HSL) starts to break down the triglyceride into a molecule called one glycerol molecule and three fatty acid molecules,

These fatty acids molecules then spread into blood and are absorbed by body tissues. Now since the glucose level fall and fatty acids level rises in the blood cells so the liver produces a compound called Acetyl-CoA.

Now the process of ketogenesis process starts and it starts to form ketones bodies. these ketones are converted into two other types of ketones called beta-hydroxybutyrate,and acetone. On the other side the glycerol of the fat molecules gets converted into glucose. and this process is termed as gluconeogenesis, also known as "making new sugar".

Now as the ketones quantity rises in the body so the heart and the brain start to use the ketones to fuel itself.

Side Effects of Ketogenic Diet:

when you start to implement low carb diet you may suffer from these types of sides effects which is perfectly normal and are manageable. Most of these side effects are temporary and can be kept under control if you know why it causes them.

In this section you will learn different types of side effects caused by ketogenic diet and steps to be taken to keep it under control. However after several weeks these side effects fades away and becomes normal

Urination:

when you start ketogenic diet or any other type of low carb diet, you will start to notice that you urinate more often than before. this urination is normal and can be coped up with by taking sodium in your daily diet. When your body is in ketogenic diet the liver goes through the process of glycogenic state meaning the liver starts to make a lot of glucose which in turn makes lots of water. As the carb intake and glycogen store drop and our kidney start to excrete lots of water in the process.

Dizziness and fatigue:

As more water is lost from the body, the minerals like salt,potassium, and magnesium become rare in your body so you will feel weak and tired and also lightheaded and dizzy.

Fatigue and dizziness are the most common side effects of the ketogenic diet . these side effects can be avoided by eating more salts or potassium rich food. Foods like

green leafy vegetables, avocados are rich in potassium and should be included in your daily diet. As long as your carb intake is lower than 60 carbs a day, you need to take more amount of salt. If you are having blood pressure issues then you should consult your doctor.

Also, it is advised to take at least 400mg of magnesium citrate before sleeping at night. However, you should consult your doctor if you are having heart and kidneys issues. It is also important to take at least 2 cups of raw green leafy vegetables every day.

Low Blood Sugar:

During a ketogenic diet, you may suffer from low blood sugar levels. This is perfectly normal and will become normal after few weeks of low carb intake. Eating 1-2 glucose tablet is the easiest and fastest way to recover from this. always carry some glucose tablet along with you whenever you travel.

Headaches:

Due to the mineral loss during the ketogenic diet, you may suffer from headaches and mild flu-like symptoms. Drink a quarter spoon of salt with water and you should feel well after few minutes. Always increase your salt and water intake and you will become normal within 3-4 days.

Constipation:

This is most common side effects when you are in low carb diet. It happens due to the salt loss and dehydration. Taking 400 mg of magnesium citrate will help to cope up with this issue. Drinking lots of water and consuming dairy products will also help you to recover from this condition. Also if you are consuming too many nuts then cut the consumption of nuts, it will make you feel better.

Sugar Cravings:

Sugar craving is another side effect of ketogenic diet, initially, you will crave sugar a lot during the low carb diet, This will happen for few weeks as the body is still under the transition stage due to which you will crave sugar and you will more likely to eat sugar. But you need to stop this compulsion of sugar cravings as it may bring back the high carb effect.

Make sure to replace the carbs with more fat.

Saturated fats like butter or coconut oil will reduce this effect. Also having a teaspoon dose of sugar-free Metamucil or plain psyllium husk powder right before the meal will also reduce the effect of craving.

Weakness:

This results due to the loss of a mineral level in your body. However, adding some more protein will recover this side effects. having a 1/4 teaspoon of salt in a glass of water will also help. You can also take 1-2 potassium citrate supplements but not more than 99 mg of it. It is advised to have potassium rich food in this case.

Muscle Cramps:

This is another side effect and it happens due to the loss of essential minerals particularly magnesium. One of the great physicians(Name not known) suggests to take at least 3 magnesium tablets such as Slow-Mag or Mag 64 for at least 20 days. However, if you have kidney problems or kidney failures then it is advised to consult the doctor before taking oral medicine.

Sleep Disturbances:

Loss of sleep in the ketogenic diet is caused due to the result of low serotonin and low insulin level. A solution of a snack which contains both protein and some carbohydrate before sleeping at night will make this symptom go away. Also, there is histamine intolerance since in low carb diet there is higher level of histamine which results in anxiety and loss of sleep.

Heart Racing issues:

If a person has low blood pressure then, he may experience heart racing or heart palpitations, this is a temporary effect and can be recovered by taking enough salt, magnesium and potassium in quantity. Try not to take tablets instead try to consume rich food containing salt, magnesium, and potassium,

Many people report that they are allergic to food like coconut oil. so try to take small amounts of this and increase it overtime, Don't rely on MTC oil for the fat intake only. Include other fat like butter,ghee, olive oil, and some animal fats also.

Also, try adding adequate protein as for some people it is necessary to have high protein intake. Try adding 10 grams of protein at each meal.

Hair Loss:

Some people report that they experience hair loss issues when they are in the ketogenic diet. However, this effect is not common in most people as hair loss can be caused by any major change in diet. Medical professionals claim that the hair loss is caused due to the change in hormone level also. As ketogenic diet lowers insulin level in the body so this may also result in hair loss issues. However, if you are having hair loss during the ketogenic diet then do not worry, because this is not permanent. this hair loss issue will revert back to time as you go through the diet for 2-3 weeks of time.

As you can see above the ketogenic diet has some side effects but these side-effects are temporary and can be controlled by applying certain strategies.

Benefits of ketogenic Diet:

The ketogenic diet can fix the hypoglycemia and sugar cravings. Ketogenic diet can control the over eating habits and is one of the most empowering benefits of ketogenic diet plan. Many people have reported that the ketogenic diet has fixed the over eating habit of sugar cravings.

Lack of Hunger- If you are struggling with food eating addiction or overeating then ketogenic diet can helpful. Sometimes you will notice that you even forget to eat food during the ketogenic diet.

Lower blood pressure. Low carb diet specially ketogenic diet are helpful in lowering blood pressure . However, if you are taking medication for blood pressure then you may feel little dizzy at the beginning stage. Talk to your doctor regarding lowering your medication dose under these circumstances.

Helps in lowering of Cholesterol: It is one of the another benefits of the ketogenic diet , as cholesterol is made up of excess glucose in the daily diet. And when you implement the ketogenic diet then you lower the chances of arterial damage and also the inflammation drastically drops. As a consequence, the cholesterol drops drastically. since the body has less glucose to make the cholesterol.

A drop in triglycerides- triglycerides is the measure of carbohydrates consumption if you are on the ketogenic diet then the level of triglycerides level drops, as a result, the risk of heart attack will drop dramatically.

Your energy level increases: If you are suffering from muscle pain then you can recover from the muscle pain easily when you are on the ketogenic diet. Your energy level increases, also if there are chronic fatigue symptoms then it will get better.

Clearer thinking: Our brain is 60% weight by fat, the more you eat fat the better it will function. Scientific evidence shows that due to an essential fatty acids the brain works properly, As a result, you are able to think clearly.

Weight Loss- Ketogenic diet is helpful in normalizing your body weight. This is a diet which can bring you the desired result with your body weight.

In this book, we will primarily discuss how you can lose weight by applying the ketogenic diet.

Digestion-your digestion will get better with the ketogenic diet plan a decrease in stomach pain, bloating, gas etc fades away and is very good for your belly.

Mood Stabilization- the ketone bodies are very beneficial in stabilizing the dopamine levels and serotonin level, as a result, helps in maintaining the better mood.

Ketogenic Diet Plan:

Before we go into the nuts and bolts of Ketogenic Diet Plan you need to know if you can apply the ketogenic diet plan.

Here are some of the medical conditions, in which one should not follow the ketogenic diet plan. Make sure to consult your doctor if you have any questions regarding the health issues you are having before going for the ketogenic diet,

List of medical conditions which is not suitable for ketogenic diet plan:

- Carnitine deficiency (primary)
- Carnitine palmitoyltransferase (CPT) I or II deficiency
- Carnitine translocase deficiency

- Beta-oxidation defects
- Mitochondrial 3-hydroxy-3-methylglutaryl-CoA synthase (mHMGS) deficiency
- Medium-chain acyl dehydrogenase deficiency (MCAD)
- Long-chain acyl dehydrogenase deficiency (LCAD)
- Short-chain acyl dehydrogenase deficiency (SCAD)
- Long-chain 3-hydroxyacyl-CoA deficiency
- Medium-chain 3-hydroxyacyl-CoA deficiency
- Pyruvate carboxylase deficiency
- Porphyria
- History of pancreatitis
- Active gall bladder disease
- Impaired liver function
- Impaired fat digestion
- Poor nutritional status
- Gastric bypass surgery
- Abdominal tumors
- Decreased gastrointestinal motility; this may be in conjunction with conventional cancer treatment and associated drugs
- History of kidney failure
- Pregnancy and lactation

NOTE: It is advised to take your doctor's advice before applying ketogenic diet plan.

Ketogenic Diet Plan

Follow these steps before applying the ketogenic diet plan.

1. First, determine your Ideal body weight. You can use the standard weight calculator to measure your Ideal body weight. You can also use the website to measure your Ideal body weight.
2. Maintaining your daily weight before taking applying the Ketogenic Diet. You can use this website to calculate the daily

determined calorie amount you should have to maintain the normal body weight. Visit this website to determine the daily calorie amount.

3.   Use the guide below to find out the amount of protein, carbohydrate, and fat based on your weight and calories calculated in step 1 and 2.

Protein Requirement: Protein should be between 1 grams to 1.5 grams Per Kilogram body mass.

Example: If a person has a body weight of 140 pounds and lean body mass of 90 pounds

To calculate the average protein intake first we need to convert the pounds into kilograms.

As, 1 pound =2.2 kilograms

So 90 pounds =90/2.2 kilograms=40.90 Kilogram.

Then multiplying 40.90 x 1 = 40.90 grams of protein

and again multiplying 40.90x 1.5= 61.63 grams of protein

So we can see from our calculation that, the average protein intake for this person would be between 40.90 to 61.63 grams per day.

Carb requirement guide:

As a general rule of thumb, 30 grams of carbohydrates per day is enough to lose weight on a ketogenic diet plan.

Fat requirement guide: How to calculate fat required during the ketogenic diet:

To calculate the fat requirement for ketogenic diet plan you need to follow the example .

Say for instance a person is over weight and has a weight of 150 pounds, he wants to gain his ideal weight, and he has decided on the daily calorie intake of 1800 calorie per day, 30 grams of carbs and 1 gram/kilogram of ideal body weight of protein.

Then we can see,

Protein: 150/2.2 = 68 kilograms = 68 x 1 gram = 68 grams or 272 calories.

Carb: 30 grams = 120 calories

Total calories from above: 272+120 = 392 calories

Fat : 1800 total calories -39 protein and carb calories = 1408fat calories

To get in grams divide fat calories by 9:

1408/9=156g of fat per day.

Food to eat during Ketogenic diet plan when you are hungry:

- Meat: beef, lamb, goat.
- Pork of any kind, but be careful with added sugar.
- Poultry: chicken, turkey, quail, goose, pheasant.
- Fish or seafood of any kind: anchovies, bass, calamari, catfish, cod, flounder, halibut, herring, mackerel, salmon, sardines, scallops, accord, sole, snapper, trout, and tuna.

- Do not use canned items as it may contain added sugar.
- Whole eggs
- Bacon and Sausage : Not more than 2 grams per servings.
- Avoid whey protein and foods until you reach weight loss goal.

No flour, breading or cornmeal protein is allowed.

Eat one to two cups of salad greens every day .

- Cabbage
- Chives
- Lettuce
- Parsley
- Kale
- Parsley
- Chard

Fibrous Vegetables

1 cup a day.

- Alfalfa and bean sprouts
- Asparagus
- Bamboo shoots
- Bell pepper
- Bok choy
- Broccoli
- Brussels sprouts
- Cucumber
- Green beans (string beans)
- Mushrooms
- Okra
- Radishes
- Rhubarb
- Snow Peas
- Summer squash
- Tomatoes
- Turnip
- Wax beans
- Water Chestnuts
- Zucchini

- Tomatoes are rich in sugar so eat raw not more than half cup.

Fat recommendations:

For cooking and heating:

- Beef tallow, from grass, fed only
- Butter, get organic only
- Chicken fat, organic only
- Duck fat, organic only
- Ghee with butter and milk solids removed
- Olive oil (organic only)
- Organic coconut oil
- Organic red palm oil in small amounts

Fat to use as Cold Dressing

- Avocado oil
- Maccdilia oil
- Seed only nuts oils: Almond oil, sesame oil, etc. Do not heat them and also limit the amount as is rich in omega 6 fatty acids
- Avoid vegetable oils completely.

Foods to eat in limited quantity:

Cheese: not more than 4 ounce per day.

- carb count must me less than 1 gram per serving
- Hard, aged cheese like Swiss and cheddar
- Soft such as Bire, Camembert, blue, mozzarella and goat cheese
- Whipped and block cream cheese with no added whey,
- Avoid processed cheeses like Velveeta and high carb types like Gjetost

Dairy Cream: not more than 4 tablespoon per day

- Heavy cream, whipping cream, or sour cream.
- Avoid half -n-half milk, also avoid labeled products.

Fatty vegetables

- Olives up to 7 a day only

- Avocado but only half per day.

Mayonnaise: not more than 4 tablespoons per day

- Less than 1 carb per serving
- Use only Duke and Hellmann brand only
- Check the label for other brands and make sure to use only those brands which have low-carb in them.

Other Condiments:

- Lime juice only 4 teaspoons/day
- Ketchup only 1 tablespoon er day
- Soy Sauces: Up to 4 tablespoon per day and uses only low carb.
- Salad dressings: Make you own with the use of oil and vinegar.
- Pickles: Check the label for the carbohydrate content and serving size. Use Bubblies brand as it is sugar-free

- Use artificial sweeteners like spices and stevia in small quantity.

Snacks:

- Pork rinds, not more than 2 servings per day
- Nuts and nut flours, not more than 1 ounce per day.
- Avoid snacks made from whey protein. It spikes insulin and hunger level.

Beverages

- Almond milk, not sweet only 2 cups/day
- Clear broth or bouillon
- Decaf coffee
- Decaf tea(unsweetened)
- Herbal tea(unsweetened)
- Water
- Flavored seltzer water (unsweetened)

Conclusion

Now you have learned the basics of ketogenic diet, now you can apply these principles to apply ketogenic diet for yourself and if you follow the plan for at least 4 weeks then you will see a drastic improvement in your weight loss.

If you found this short book helpful then you can leave your review on Amazon here---->> https://www.amazon.com/dp/B01M0D9GCV